Telemedicine

A Practical Guide for Professionals-

2021 New Edition

Andrea Kamenca, MBA

MINDVIEW PRESS

Oregon City, Oregon

For all of the people working to create telemedicine services for the benefit of patients. You are making a difference! Thank you.

TABLE OF CONTENTS

Author's Note- 2021

When I wrote the first edition of this book, I didn't anticipate more than 1200 people purchasing it, nor did I predict a pandemic changing everything. My original intention was to write a practical, brief text for the students in my Arizona State University graduate school telemedicine class. I am grateful and humbled to know my book has also been used by professionals who are actively deploying telemedicine.

The purpose of this book remains the same, to provide you, the professional, an overview of telemedicine. This new edition, updated with COVID-19 specific information, is still meant to serve as an implementation guide should you desire to stand up telemedicine in your hospital, practice, or facility. It is NOT an exhaustive text. However, this new edition nearly doubles the active links in the text and appendices. Please use the 150+ links! I chose them for their quality and relevance.

I entered the healthcare field working for a specialized public health clinic. During that time, a respected healthcare leader introduced me to telemedicine. I spent the next four years implementing a host of telemedicine projects for multiple organizations. I found significant knowledge gaps, especially when implementing and scaling a telemedicine program.

One of the few silver linings of the COVID-19 pandemic has been the widespread adoption of telemedicine and its entry into the mainstream. As clinicians have struggled to reduce infections, treat COVID-19, and manage other chronic conditions, telemedicine has proven the optimum solution. Finally, primary care physicians, hospitals, and specialists are routinely using it.

And, finally, with changes by the Centers for Medicare and Medicaid (CMS), getting paid for telemedicine encouraged clinicians to use it as a viable option for seeing patients. People afraid to use technology to see their doctor seemed to diminish.

When I wrote the book's first edition, I was deeply disappointed in the lack of telemedicine adoption. I wish it hadn't taken a pandemic to make it happen, but here we are. The first book helped doctors and clinicians to understand telemedicine better. It also served as a supplemental text to the Arizona State University Telemedicine course in the Bioinformatics program. The second edition will, as well. The second edition will update the information and expand sections, explicitly addressing the impact and changes relevant to the COVID-19 pandemic.

Telemedicine has tremendous promise to make our health system more personal and practical. It is more likely to be successful when a devoted team thoughtfully and consistently addresses the organizational and operational details required to make the projects a clinical reality. Telemedicine will be successful when planned, piloted, launched, and scaled like other clinical systems.

Healthcare professionals are busy. It is tough to get "mind share" for innovation. It is complicated to make a case for new delivery methods, like telemedicine, that may or may not include incremental revenue. Most organizations use a technology purchase to prompt the discussion or force a pilot project. Yet, these pilot projects are often unsustainable or unable to scale due to the significant operational processes not addressed during the pilot.

My goal was to provide enough information to scan the book and use it as a resource. The appendix (and text) is rich with links to federal programs, research, organizations, mailing lists, and other resources to build your knowledge base and your program. If you have any comments, feel free to send an email at andrea.innovia@gmail.com

Thank you for reading.

Andrea

Part 1 Telemedicine Foundations

Chapter 1

Telemedicine Then and Now

What is Telemedicine?

Telemedicine refers to the delivery of healthcare services via an electronic device. Examples include continuous monitoring of patients in a hospital, a consumer accessing a physician over a web camera at home for a diagnosis and a potential pharmaceutical treatment, and even the movement of images to access specialized radiologists for diagnosis. Because of the COVID-19 pandemic, patients have accessed their providers over the telephone, via a smartphone, laptop computer, or tablet. All of these can be called "telemedicine."

Telehealth is a broader term that includes providing medical care and consultations and includes education and training delivered using technology and communication systems. The broadest term is exchanging medical information from one site to another via electronic communications to provide patient care, treatment, and services. Some examples include diabetes education, grand rounds by residents, and post-operative care.

Telemedicine Then

In the beginning, rural areas used telemedicine to gain specialized physician services. Typically, they would install a complex and proprietary communications system and then reach an agreement with an urban hospital. The rural hospital physician in an emergency room, for example, would contact a stroke neurologist in a nearby urban center using those proprietary systems when potential stroke patients arrived in the emergency department.

Telemedicine funding, considered a tool for the rural areas, was distributed by federal government agencies like the Department of Agriculture and the Federal Communications Commission, not the Department of Health and Human Services, as one might expect. The proprietary systems and regional telemedicine resource centers were primarily grant-funded, and the opportunity to bill for telemedicine health services delivered depended upon rural geography. The states who pioneered Telemedicine were mostly the Western states due to the large geography and distance between rural and urban areas. States like Arizona, New Mexico, Texas, and others were creating telemedicine networks before the technology tools we enjoy today.

Telemedicine Now

Now, broadband and cellular access are ubiquitous. People are comfortable with technology. The dynamic nature of today's healthcare environment is forcing practitioners, healthcare systems, administrators, and patients to seek new, more effective care delivery methods even in urban settings. The explosive growth in the retail clinics located inside pharmacies from 2010 to 2017 proves the average patient as a consumer is willing to seek care in alternative settings. At the same time, payment for medical services is shifting from fee-for-service-based models to population health management. Telemedicine as a delivery tool not only manages population health and offers convenience to low acuity patients, it also can monitor medically complex patients, create new revenue sources, and shift the care continuum.

Although broadband and cellular are almost everywhere, the patients most likely to use the healthcare system have been the least equipped to use it. Lower-income and older patients are less likely to have the equipment and be comfortable using it. The pandemic forced the issue. People like my parents were forced to learn how to use the technology, using their children's or neighbors' help accessing services delivered via smartphones and tablets. Together, we will see how telemedicine will be adopted permanently after the pandemic. I suspect it will remain as another way to deliver care. And, large entities like Walmart and Amazon are working to deliver

Telemedicine Challenges

Before the COVID pandemic, there were several challenges surrounding telemedicine's use. Key challenges included complicated billing, cross-state licensure, state laws that vary regarding the definition of a medical exam, malpractice insurance, and a lack of trained people to implement complex telemedicine programs. Most of these challenges have been resolved. Telemedicine can be billed to your insurance, Medicaid and Medicare. (More in the finance chapter!) Telemedicine continues to grow exponentially. Hundreds of successful telemedicine implementations are making a positive difference for patients. And, the adoption of telemedicine during the pandemic may fundamentally change the landscape of how telemedicine is provided to patients experiencing chronic conditions.

COVID's Impact

The beginning of the pandemic (April 2020) showed telemedicine usage, as measured by claim volumes, increased from 78X the previous levels. By June, it reduced to "only" 38x the volume from February 2020. McKinsey and Company estimates that "up to $250 billion of US Healthcare spend could potentially be shifted to virtual or virtually enabled care."

Telemedicine is here to stay, especially for office visits and outpatient care. It seems several factors brought about this change. 1) The promotion of telemedicine by the Federal government, especially the President. President Trump was very public in his support for telemedicine. That helped the adoption. 2) Consumers are much more "wired" and have mobile phones with the bandwidth and capacity to participate in telemedicine. 3) providers were faced with the reality of patients needing their services, but the providers needed a safe way to deliver those services. 4) Important regulatory changes occurred redefining telemedicine, offering new reimbursements, and reducing regulatory requirements related to licensing.

Chapter 2

Trends Creating Telemedicine Opportunities

Before the COVID pandemic, a "perfect storm" of trends pressured existing healthcare delivery methods to change. These trends include rising medical costs, an aging population, extended life spans, an increase in complex chronic conditions, and consumerism. COVID forced the issue. Patients with chronic conditions who were at higher risk for infection wanted to avoid other potentially infected people who might be sitting in the doctor's office. And, people suffering from depression and anxiety needed a way to receive support. Telemedicine assisted with those two objectives, among others. Below is a brief overview of trends boosting telemedicine's growth.

Technology

The American Recovery and Reinvestment Act and the Health Information Technology for Economic and Clinical Health Act (HITECH Act) of 2009 offered significant incentives for hospitals to implement electronic health records (EHRs). As this tremendous shift occurred, healthcare embarked upon a new path to technology-based systems. Healthcare has been a "laggard" industry regarding its technology adoption, but the EHR implementations opened the door for additional technology solutions. The new emphasis on technology has transformed large health systems and has dramatically increased the number of technological experts available to assist with technology adoption. Subsequent legislation, including the 21st Century Cares Act, further expanded the role of technology, including provisions to improve the flow and exchange of electronic health information."

Accountability in the Acute Care Environment

The Affordable Care Act (ACA) and healthcare payment trends encouraged new payment models that emphasized prevention, population health, and a wider view of healthcare delivery. Medicare and Medicaid have paid a "fee for service" for hospital stays and procedures. Consequently, hospital costs have dramatically escalated. Medicare is trying to drive down acute care costs and is making acute environments more accountable for outcomes.

For example, Medicare withholds hospital payment for patients who, after initial hospitalization, are re-hospitalized within 30 days. At the same time, Medicare is working to align patient acuity more closely with the appropriate care setting. They are using financial pressure to shift payment from acute care to the post-acute environment.

Population Health Management, New Payment Models, and the Triple Aim

One of telemedicine's key drivers is the shift to population health management. Accountable care organizations, health maintenance organizations, and others are exploring strategies to limit medical care consumption by keeping patients healthy and encouraging the appropriate care setting for their ailment. Population health management is changing how and where healthcare is delivered.

Telemedicine delivers health care in new settings like a patient's home, much more affordable sites than the emergency department or inpatient facilities. To that end, telemedicine assists population health managers by driving down the cost of care. It offers a way to manage patients outside of the traditional care continuum, thereby saving costs and improving outcomes.

The recent changes in payment, a shift to the non-acute setting, and quality measures have prompted organizations to develop a "Triple Aim" of the targeted improvements. Developed by Don Berwick, Tom Nolan, and John Wittington, the Triple Aim measures a population's overall health, the individual patient's experience of care and, the per capita cost of care. The Triple Aim's goal is to improve a patient's health while the care experience is good and costs decrease. The Institute for Healthcare Improvement (IHI), the US National Quality Strategy, and other organizations worldwide have adopted the Triple Aim as a comprehensive goal for health systems.

Aging Population Living Longer with Chronic Conditions

The baby boom population is the largest in the United States. Born between 1944 and 1964, more than 10,000 people turn 65 years of age and are eligible for Medicare every day. Between 2000 and 2019, people aged 65 and up increased from 12.4 to 16.5%, with some states like Montana, Florida, and Hawaii already having an over-65 population between 19 and 21.2%. Maine has 21.2% of its population at or above 65 years of age. According to previous information released by the Populations Reference Bureau (PRB), in 1960, only 9% of the population was older than 65. By 2030, 21% of the population will be more than 65 years of age. In addition, they are living far longer than previous generations.

Chronic conditions are common among an aging population. As people age, chronic conditions get more complex and increase in number. Therefore, telemedicine tools like remote patient monitoring offer realistic and affordable solutions that successfully manage a population that is aging, living longer, and has multiple chronic complex conditions.

Patients with chronic conditions like diabetes and depression and those who have breathing problems or are immunocompromised are much more likely to use telemedicine in 2020. Their requirements needed treatment, and telemedicine was a way to deliver their care.

Emergency Room Use as Primary Care

Because EMTALA requires people to be treated in the emergency department regardless of their ability to pay, emergency departments are sometimes overused by people who need a primary care appointment or mental health services. Emergency departments, initially established to treat traumatic and emergent situations, are bursting at the seams. Estimates range from 3.3% to 90 percent of emergency room care is unnecessary or avoidable. Using telepsychiatry in the emergency department is viable to alleviate emergency room crowding.

Fewer Primary Care Physicians

The number of primary care physicians has steadily decreased, increasing the burden on active family care practitioners. To be successful, a family practitioner must see 20 to 24 patients per day. A typical family practice operating above capacity may not see a patient for three weeks or more. These conditions limit patients' options for managing chronic diseases, low-acuity injuries, or nuisance illnesses like colds and flu. Telemedicine is being used to treat low acuity patients and is a viable alternative for patients who cannot schedule a provider appointment. The COVID pandemic demonstrated the efficacy of telemedicine to care for acute patients who do not need an in-person appointment. Physician extenders, like Physician Assistants and Nurse Practitioners, are using telemedicine to monitor chronic patients.

Patients Less Likely to Have a Primary Care Physician

Millennials, a young, more technologically astute population, visit a variety of healthcare providers, reversing the trend of the primary care physician as the center of a family or patient's care. Estimates are that 17-42% of patients are "un-doctored," meaning they do not have a primary care physician who manages their care. In addition, they are more likely to see a doctor over a web camera whether or not they acknowledge a relationship with a family care provider. Particularly for young mothers, telemedicine is a convenient alternative to piling children into a vehicle and waiting in a doctor's office.

Patient as Consumer

Burdened with increased financial responsibility for their health care, the patient acts more like a consumer with choices and less like a patient who is provided care. Today, consumers are more likely to choose a doctor or hospital due to convenience, speed, or cost, almost as if they choose a restaurant.

About six years ago, retail pharmacies started capitalizing on this trend. The retail pharmacies discovered that patients increasingly sought care outside of the "normal" office hours physicians were keeping. They turned their brands and locations into more than just "drug stores." They built pharmacies with embedded clinics on nearly every urban corner staffed by mid-level providers like nurse practitioners and physician assistants. They are providing consumers with a lower-cost alternative to the primary care physician or urgent care.

Now, the start-up and expansion of direct-to-consumer telemedicine companies like Doctor on Demand, American Well, and Teladoc are offering a panel of physicians to provide low acuity urgent care for patients who are savvy enough to use technology to see the doctor. The people using this service are primarily working mothers. Walmart sees a future here, as well, having recently purchased Me MD.

Extending Specialists

As mentioned earlier, specialists reside primarily in urban areas. Telemedicine enables patients in rural areas to access those specialists. Yet, even urban doctors may cover multiple acute care facilities on any one given day. Rather than the doctor traveling throughout the city, telemedicine is used to conduct an initial consultation to determine if a specialist needs to drive and lay hands on the patient. At one of the large healthcare systems, they assigned an infectious disease doctor to multiple emergency rooms who could take consultations in her central, urban office. After examination, the patient required a consultation, and the physician would drive to the suburban hospital for the in-person exam.

Technology Comfort

As patients become increasingly comfortable using technology, cell phone use improves, and broadband access is available, there are lower barriers to using technology to deliver and receive medical care.

Telemedicine offers solutions to address more than a dozen trends in healthcare. Telemedicine enables providers to deliver specialty care to patients regardless of location, assist with chronic disease management, provide continuous monitoring of in-hospital, rural, or home-bound patients, and improve the patient experience by offering convenience, connection, and access to care. Patients benefit due to the convenience, reduced cost, and improved care. Telemedicine has great promise.

COVID's Impact

Prior to COVID-19, people needed to learn the video component in order to participate in a telehealth visit. It was required in order to bill for the visit. That said, the frequent users of healthcare are often patients who are tech-averse, lack access to technology, or not tech-savvy. One of the changes made by the Center for Medicare and Medicaid (CMS) was to allow telephone calls without video to "count" as video visits. Further, those in rural areas may lack broadband access or the required infrastructure to support telemedicine. The Department of Health and Human Services has significantly expanded the support for rural areas. They also instituted flexible provisions to support telemedicine in rural areas. Some of the provisions include:

- They are offering HIPAA flexibility to employ commonly used apps, not currently compliant with HIPAA rules. These apps include Facetime, Facebook Messenger, Zoom, Skype, and Google Hangouts.
- Telehealth waivers to allow providers to see patients in their homes and outside of rural areas, practice remote care, deliver care for both established and new patients, and BILL for telehealth visits as if they were provided in person.
- Temporary expansion of telehealth services allowing Federally Qualified Health Centers and Rural Health Clinics to offer telemedicine services from their site and to patients' homes. They also allow emergency room visits, nursing facility and discharge

visits, home visits, and therapy services to be covered via telehealth.

- They are allowing providers to reduce or waive cost-sharing for telehealth and other virtual care paid for by federal programs like Medicare, Medicaid, and the Children's Health Insurance Program (CHIP) during a health emergency.

Many private insurers peg their reimbursements to CMS allowable reimbursements. Consequently, many private insurers have allowed medical providers to bill telemedicine visits like they would in-person visits. It is difficult to predict what will be allowable after the pandemic recedes to manageable levels. But, certainly, the unprecedented use of telemedicine is here to stay.

Chapter 3

Telemedicine Concepts and Definitions

Telemedicine offers myriad applications and uses. Like most unique and complex fields, telemedicine has developed a lexicon of terms. Although countless terms may apply to telemedicine, this section reviews the most common.

Terms sometimes used interchangeably are Telehealth and telemedicine. Yet, there is a distinct difference between the two terms. Specifically, telehealth is the exchange of medical information between one site and another with the objective of providing medical care, consultation, or education using information technology. Telehealth is a broader term than telemedicine.

Telemedicine is a subset of telehealth. Specifically, the definition of telemedicine is medical care enabled by the use of information technology between a medical provider in one physical location and a medical provider or patient in another physical location.

Telemedicine includes patient monitoring. Patient monitoring can occur at the patient's home or in an acute setting, like the intensive care unit. The concept of patient monitoring includes continuous monitoring and remote patient monitoring. Continuous monitoring assesses a patient's condition by tracking the patient's medical data. Including continuous monitoring under the umbrella of telemedicine means one must incorporate the viewing of a patient through a camera or other technology to assess their condition. One example is eICU, a Philips program that monitors patient's vitals and other medical data while the patient is in the ICU.

Whereas remote patient monitoring includes the use of devices to track and report health conditions in an outpatient setting. Typically, remote patient monitoring occurs in the home of patients, with the medical data sent to their health care provider for review and follow-up.

Identifying the type of telemedicine transaction is critical to billing for the service and defines the type of telemedicine encounter. The two kinds of telemedicine encounters are asynchronous, meaning not occurring at the same time and, synchronous or occurring simultaneously in "real-time." An asynchronous or "Store and Forward" example is a photo of a dermatological condition sent to a dermatologist for later assessment and diagnosis. A synchronous encounter, for example, is a video consultation between a patient in a rural emergency department and a stroke neurologist in an urban location.

Telemedicine programs between urban and rural areas have developed their language. Sometimes called the Hub and Spoke arrangement, the "Hub" refers to a central location, usually in an urban area, where physician experts reside. The "Spoke sites" are rural or community hospitals that are served by the hub site. Another term for the "spoke site" is "distant site," whereas the urban location is called the "originating site."

With the advent of mobile devices, telemedicine services delivered via mobile devices are sometimes labeled mHealth, eHealth, digital health, or virtual health. Most of these terms refer to the use of mobile technology and wireless devices to improve health outcomes, deliver healthcare services and health research.(HIMSS)

Chapter 4

Telemedicine Types and Categories

Telemedicine is more than a patient “seeing” a physician over a web camera. The definition is much broader. The first step in determining if telemedicine is right for your organization is deciding the type of telemedicine to pilot and explore. There are many distinctive types of telemedicine. Telemedicine service categories are roles of the people participating in the clinical interaction, and the setting of services offered, and transaction timing. This chapter describes the various types of telemedicine services and their categories.

Provider to Provider (P2P)

A P2P consultation occurs between physicians or providers. The interaction can occur synchronously or asynchronously. For example, a surgeon consulting with an oncologist using a live video feed is a provider-to-provider telemedicine encounter. Another example is an emergency physician consulting with a specialist without the patient being present.

Provider to Consumer (P2C)

A provider-to-patient or provider to "consumer" encounter is a face-to-face encounter between a provider and a patient via a web camera, robot, cart, or other video technology. The encounter occurs regardless of patient location, acuity level, or payer and can occur synchronously or asynchronously. It also includes continuous monitoring of patients with a visual monitoring device like a camera in the Intensive care unit or NICU.

Provider to Provider to Consumer (P2P2C)

The provider-to-provider-to-consumer interaction involves consultation between physicians or providers while incorporating the patient into the interaction. Examples include emergency room psychiatric consultation requested by the emergency room physician with the psychiatrist evaluating the patient while present in the emergency department and a stroke neurologist examining the patient. In contrast, the emergency room physician is present during the video encounter.

Training: Provider to Provider and Educator to Consumer

Telehealth versus telemedicine includes education and the dissemination of health information. Although this book does not elaborate on these encounters, these examples are valuable applications in the telehealth field. Telehealth offerings can include medical education (CME, Tumor Boards, ECHO Model), consumer health information (Patients Like Me, WebMD, Patient Portal, Self-Monitoring Devices), and consumer medical information (Diabetes Education, Wound Dressing, First Aid.)

Telemedicine Setting (Acute versus Ambulatory)

Another way to categorize telemedicine is to consider the setting in which it is utilized. Telemedicine can occur in the acute environment, like the emergency department, the intensive care unit, the neonatal ICU, or even the surgical suite.

Alternatively, it can occur in the ambulatory, home, and skilled nursing settings. When considering telemedicine, it is crucial to consider the setting, as it affects the billing and operational details associated with delivering the care.

Synchronous v Asynchronous

Categorizing types of telemedicine encounters as synchronous, i.e. occurring simultaneously or asynchronous, meaning there is a separation between the medical event and the diagnosis, is another method for categorizing telemedicine encounters.

Summary Chart

The chart below lists telemedicine use-case examples and their categories.

Type of Telemedicine service	Type of telemedicine service	Setting	Synchro nous /Asynch ronous
ICU / NICU monitoring	Continuous Monitoring or Provider to Consumer	Acute	S
Telestroke Networks, Behavioral Health	Provider to provider to consumer	Acute, Ambulatory	S
Dermatology, Pathology	Provider to provider	Acute or Ambulatory	A
Internal medicine doctor discusses case with cardiologist	Provider to provider consults	Acute or Ambulatory	S
Tumor Boards, Grand Rounds, Project Echo	Medical Education	Acute or Ambulatory	S, A
Chronic Complex patient visits	Provider to existing patient	Ambulatory	S
Various companies including	Provider to new patient (on demand)	Ambulatory, Occupational Health	S

Teladoc, American Well, Doctor on Demand			
Post-Discharge CHF patients monitored	Home monitoring	Ambulatory	S
Radiology images read by radiologists	Image Sharing	Acute and Ambulatory	A

Part 2 Telemedicine Examples

Chapter 5

Prominent Uses of Telemedicine

Telestroke

Telestroke is the most prevalent and popular use of telemedicine. Stroke symptoms require immediate assessment and intervention. When an ischemic stroke is diagnosed within four hours of onset and a “clot-busting” drug administered, the likelihood of permanent disability and death significantly diminishes. If there is no neurologist on-site, telestroke, a type of telemedicine service, facilitates the stroke diagnosis process by connecting emergency physicians with distant stroke neurologists within the critical window of time. Whether an urban health system offers a hub and spoke model or rural entities contract with stand-alone physician organizations for telestroke services, telestroke services increase the likelihood that someone will fully recover from a stroke.

There are many telestroke programs in the United States. You can find examples of telestroke programs by contacting the American Health Association and the American Stroke Association. Many telestroke programs have a close relationship with the tPA pharmaceutical manufacturer, Genentech.

Telestroke is one of the few telemedicine programs that require specific and reliable technology. For the most part, technology is the least important aspect of telemedicine. Many types of software and hardware can be used effectively. InTouch is the industry leader for telestroke technology and maintains an exceptional response time, as well as "uptime" for its technology. Although it is costly, it is widely acknowledged that it is very reliable! When "time is brain," "uptime" or reliability is critical to a fast and reliable response time.

Telepsychiatry

Telepsychiatry solves persistent and recurring problems in healthcare. Namely,

•One in eight visits to the emergency department is psychiatry-related
•There is a shortage of in-patient beds
•There are 4000 health professional shortage areas
•There are only 28,000 psychiatrists, nationwide
•Telepsychiatry can improve ED throughput, result in fewer in-patient admissions.

Given these statistics, it is not surprising that telepsychiatry is the second most utilized type of telemedicine in the United States.

More than four thousand mental health professional shortage areas are identified across the United States. In many areas of the country, a patient in a psychiatric crisis has only one option: the local Emergency Department.

The use of emergency room telepsychiatry benefits hospitals by supporting faster psychiatric consults improved ED throughput, and in some areas, the ability to lift or place involuntary psychiatric holds. Therefore, telepsychiatry in the emergency department can cause fewer inpatient admissions, better patient and staff satisfaction, and earlier diagnosis and therapy.

The use of telepsychiatry in an outpatient setting can mean more patients are getting more convenient and accessible care. They can obtain psychiatric services at a clinic or even in the privacy of their homes.

Low Acuity Urgent Care

Low acuity urgent care visits, also named video visits, eVisits, virtual visits, or teleurgent care, are defined as provider-to-consumer telemedicine services where the consumer or patient uses a computer, telephone, or mobile device to participate in a clinical consultation using a computer or device webcam, telephone or via email. A prescription or referral is often generated.

Like Walgreens and CVS, retail pharmacies discovered that patients were seeking care outside of the “normal” business hours physicians were keeping. They turned their brands into healthcare centers and built facilities on nearly every corner in urban areas. They provided the consumer with an alternative to the primary care physician, urgent care provider, and emergency department visit. The pharmacies discovered that:

• 7% of adults visited the emergency room due to a lack of access to other providers.
•48% went to the emergency room because the doctor’s office was not open.
•43% of people do not have access to same or next-day PCP appointments.

Further, as the patient increasingly shoulders the cost of healthcare visits, they are shopping for lower-cost alternatives to urgent care and the family physician.

Typically, in the United States, the average cost of primary care provider visit is $131, urgent care visit is

$163, and an Emergency Department visit is $1477 (8%)

Nontraditional healthcare providers like Teladoc, American Well, and Doctor on Demand have developed teleurgent care services for the time-pressed and technology fluent healthcare consumer. More recently, Amazon and Walmart have developed or purchased providers to invest heavily in low acuity urgent care.

Insurers and accountable care organizations (ACOs) are working to drive down the cost of care. Because the average telemedicine call costs $40-50, insurers and accountable care organizations are realizing savings of $79-1427 per visit as the telemedicine visit replaces other settings. By some estimates, in 2018, teleurgent care visits are already exceeding 1.2 million annually, resulting in significant savings. That may be part of the reason insurers are purchasing telemedicine companies, like Cigna purchasing MD Live.

Chapter 6

Teleradiology

Teleradiology is an example of an asynchronous service that has gained popularity in the last ten years. Teleradiology is the movement of medical images, including digital x-rays, MRI, ultrasound, CT scan, and nuclear medicine studies, from one site to another in order to be viewed, reviewed, interpreted, or analyzed by a radiologist.

Teleradiology programs are used by hospitals and even radiology practices to cover overnight radiology shifts, acquire the specialized services of subspecialty radiologists, and cover gaps in regular radiology staffing.

Teleradiology services are proving to be a revenue generator for hospitals with significant bench strength of subspecialty physicians. They are creating teleradiology programs offering the services of their subspecialty physicians to hospitals, insurance companies, and other organizations that need a first or second opinion.

Tele Skilled Nursing Facility

Skilled Nursing Facilities and other care settings throughout the care continuum are investigating innovative ways to improve outcomes, reduce costs, and enhance the patient experience. Telehealth is a powerful tool to assist physicians with clinical assessment and accurate diagnosis while extending their oversight across multiple sites.

Typically, fewer physicians are managing more patients in the skilled nursing environment than in a hospital setting. Nurses or medical assistants provide most of the care. They call the doctor when a change of condition occurs and offer a verbal description of the situation. A report by the Kaiser Family Foundation found that 30 to 67 percent of hospitalizations among SNF residents could be prevented with well-targeted interventions. Telehealth is one of those interventions.

Opioid Substance Use/Abuse Treatments

The widespread opioid use and often stealth abuse problem plaguing this nation has created an opportunity for treatment via telemedicine. Using telemedicine allows patients the privacy to be treated in the privacy of their homes. One study has shown medical-assisted treatment programs (MAT) are equally effective via telemedicine or in-person. The Federal government agrees.

Endocrinology and Diabetes Treatment

According to a Kaiser Family Foundation white paper regarding the impact of the COVID-19 pandemic on the use of telemedicine, telediabetes care grew significantly. Further research and study showed a greater "mean reduction in hemoglobin A1c" when patients were managed using telemedicine. The CDC cites 13% of all US adults had diabetes in 2018. There are an estimated 34.5% of US adults with prediabetes. Worldwide, the rates are rising exponentially, as well.

Fertility

Specialists in the field of fertility may find an additional revenue stream, as well as helping patients outside of a close geographical area. Washington University Physicians proves this use case is viable.

School-Based Telehealth

The Kansas University Medical Center has made significant strides in offering telemedicine services to children in rural areas. Called Telehealth ROCKS (Rural Outreach for the Children of Kansas) Schools, the program offers children and school nurses a way to see family practitioners. Program providers are working with Project ECHO to gain telemedicine skills.

High-Risk Maternity

An important double-blind placebo-controlled study using telemedicine for women with high-risk pregnancies found significantly better outcomes and lower costs for women than the control group.

Monitoring Inpatient Outcomes in the ICU

Offsite intensivists now monitor about 10 percent of all critical care patients, and the results have been rewarding. Banner Health's eICU program has saved lives while reducing costs and preserving resources. The program is run from a central operations center staffed with critical care doctors and nurses. These providers remotely monitor more than 600 ICU beds in more than 25 hospitals in seven Western states, providing welcome clinical support to hospital staff. Since launching the program, Banner Health ICUs are reporting some of the lowest ICU mortality rates in the country. In 2014, Banner Health reduced predicted ICU days by 20,000, saved $68 million, and saved an estimated 2,000 lives.

Monitoring the Tiniest of Patients

Multiple health systems promote the benefits associated with teleneonatal monitoring, including positive outcomes for the baby and attachment between child and parent. Utah Valley Regional Medical Center in Provo, Utah, collaborated with

VSee, to support the 60-bed NICU. The system provides two-way communication between physicians and parents. What's more, families can access a live stream of their baby 24/7, which helps them stay connected between visits.

Monitoring Patients with Complex Chronic Illness at Home

Studies have shown remote patient monitoring reduces unnecessary emergency department usage by 25–50 percent. Several models have proven to be beneficial, including 1)Providing patients with CHF, COPD, and other chronic conditions with remote monitoring devices to track their vital signs and symptoms; 2)Care coordinators monitoring the medications and vital signs of people with limited social support; 3) Monitoring patients post-discharge to improve outcomes, medication compliance, and reduce preventable readmissions.

This chapter lists just a few of the possible telemedicine programs and projects. Telemedicine is being used by emergency services personnel, in prisons, on oil rigs, by the military, and in catastrophic conditions. The possibilities are far-reaching and quite promising. Other types of telemedicine uses include Tele-

Audiology
Cardiology
Chaplaincy
Dentistry
Dermatology
Infectious disease
Nursing
Ophthalmology
Pathology
Pharmacy
Rehabilitation
Surgery
Thoracic
Trauma Care

Chapter 7

A Special Program: Project Echo

Project ECHO, located at the University of New Mexico, initiated by Dr. Sanjeev Arora, connects specialists in population centers with providers in areas that do not have access to medical specialists. The program is enabled by telehealth technology and endeavors to "demonopolize specialty knowledge" in medicine.

"The ECHO model® links expert specialist teams at an academic 'hub' with primary care clinicians in local communities – the 'spokes' of the model. Together, they participate in weekly teleECHO® clinics, like virtual grand rounds, combined with mentoring and patient case presentations. During teleECHO clinics, primary care clinicians from multiple sites present patient cases to the specialist teams and to each other, discuss new developments relating to their patients, and determine treatment. Specialists serve as mentors and colleagues, sharing their medical knowledge and expertise with primary care clinicians. Essentially, ECHO® creates ongoing learning communities where primary care clinicians receive support and develop the skills they need to treat a particular condition." (Arora, 2013)

"Project ECHO started as a way to meet local healthcare needs. Sanjeev Arora, M.D., a liver disease doctor in Albuquerque, was frustrated that thousands of New Mexicans with hepatitis C could not get the treatment they needed because there were no specialists where they lived. The clinic where he worked was one of only two in the entire state that treated hepatitis C.

The ECHO model®, launched in 2003, makes specialized medical knowledge accessible wherever it is needed to save and improve people's lives. By putting local clinicians together with specialist teams at academic medical centers in weekly virtual clinics or teleECHO® clinics, Project ECHO shares knowledge and expands treatment capacity. The result is better care for more people.

Treatment for hepatitis C is now available at centers of excellence across New Mexico, and more than 3,000 doctors, nurses, and community health workers provide treatment to more than 6,000 patients enrolled in Project ECHO's comprehensive disease management programs for myriad conditions." (Arora, 2015)

Project ECHO operates more than 203 hubs in the US, 423 global hubs, and 920 ECHO programs in 44 countries.

Project ECHO's COVID response has been robust! Between February 3, 2020, and July 25, 2021, There have been 14,982 organizations, 8,366 sessions, 879 programs, and 1,107,780 people in attendance learning how to use telemedicine to treat people using telemedicine. They were uniquely positioned to provide guidance in the United States for Nursing Homes via the AHRQ ECHO National Nursing Home COVID-19 Action Network program and to treat the indigenous peoples in the US. Across the world, they collaborated with the WHO to lead responses in Africa, Brazil, India, and other countries.

Robert Wood Johnson, in 2009, awarded Project ECHO a prestigious, $5 million Pioneer award to expand the program and have since funded additional program expansions.

Additional Project ECHO funders include Bristol Myers Squibb, General Electric Foundation, Helmsley Charitable Trust, Con Alma Health Foundation, McCune Foundation, State of New Mexico, the Department of Defense, and federal entities, AHRQ, CDC, CMS, DoD, VA, NIDA, and the NIH.

Part 3 Building a Program

Chapter 8

Creating the Program Structure

Organizations faced with launching telemedicine at the beginning of the pandemic may have scrambled to find solutions and education to quickly stand up telemedicine functionality. New and sometimes temporary processes were employed. Once the pandemic recedes to manageable levels, providers may want to capitalize on this "new" way to see patients. To do so, approach the new offering as one would any complex program. Some hastily made decisions may need to be reversed, especially when the DHHS waivers expire. These waivers are currently allowing healthcare providers to use non-HIPAA compliant technologies to see patients.

If you have decided to start, change, or expand a telemedicine program, it is essential to develop a program structure. This section will elaborate upon more critical aspects of building a program, like creating a business plan, understanding billing, and choosing technology. Overall, telemedicine program development should include the following steps:

Build a Foundation by Creating Vision, Strategy, and Goals

First, determine your vision for the telemedicine program. What are you trying to accomplish? Are you exploring its uses? Are you trying to solve a specific problem? Are you looking for new ways to engage with patients? Is it a way to reduce overcrowding in the emergency department?

Once you have determined your vision, create a strategy for success. That strategy should include executive sponsorship, clinician support, and a budget. It could consist of a small pilot or a significant go-live.

Establish the goals associated with the vision and the strategy. For example, do you want people to use it? How much use would be considered "project success?” On the other hand, is the goal to gather information for future deployment? As is advisable in other projects, clearly stating the vision, strategy (or mission), and goals will increase success. When establishing the goals, also incorporate the metrics that will be used to measure progress.

Expand the Foundation with Budget, Governance, Reporting

Make a financial commitment to the program’s success, at least during the pilot phase. Without a budget, your telemedicine project will be a secondary research endeavor only.

Once you have determined your vision, created your strategy, established measurable goals, and made a financial commitment, decide the type of telemedicine that aligns with these factors. NOTE: Some people start with a telemedicine solution or technology first, but it is more likely to succeed if you set a vision, strategy, goals, and budget before choosing the telemedicine solution.

Governance is an essential aspect of program success. Formal healthcare systems have committees and forums to facilitate communication and to develop a consensus of support among leadership. Any organization attempting to launch telemedicine, even if traditional governance avenues do not exist, should consider creating an informal cross-functional committee of leaders to facilitate the project's success. Telemedicine's complexity necessitates that every aspect of the organization will be touched. Having a leadership team committed to the program's success is valuable and necessary for long-term success.

Consistently reporting the operational status and the metrics measuring its success keeps the project on track and takes the subjectivity out of the program's progress.

Choosing a Platform

Once a foundation has been built, take the time to choose a software platform and vendor with whom you can collaborate for the long term. A partnership with a vendor will contribute to a successful project. Excellent and comprehensive telemedicine software tools already exist. Do not develop a custom platform. It is a costly venture that requires long-term maintenance. Unless software development is a core competency of the organization, select a software vendor.

Create a pilot plan that limits the number of clinicians that need to be trained. Creating a successful pilot means choosing participants (including people and staff) who are flexible, open-minded, and cooperative. Ideally, they are also communicative and have a positive attitude towards innovation.

Set a go-live date and work towards that date by building your operational plans to include checklists, workflows, and data flows in conjunction with the impacted department (e.g., emergency department, surgical suite, primary care physician's office.)

Pilot Plan with Communications and Training

Develop an internal communications plan and execute. Ensure that all constituents, including the information technology department, administration, risk, quality, legal, and medical leadership, are apprised of the plan and support its success.

Develop an external communications plan. Communicating with patients can be complex. Using tools like the Flesch Kincaid tool embedded into Microsoft Word can assist with writing text applicable to a diverse patient population. Communicating with patients usually means describing the encounter, explaining how it works, gaining their agreement to participate, and allaying any fears about privacy. Telemedicine typically does not need the complex "consenting" associated with human trials but reviewing those guidelines can positively inform the communications.

Conduct training for all participants in the telemedicine pilot. Specifically, focus on the providers and staff that will be the "boots on the ground." At the elbow, training combined with job aids, workflow lists, and screen captures will improve the likelihood of success.

The day before go-live, test the equipment, notify everyone impacted, and be present for last-minute questions and issues.

Build an Enduring Program Infrastructure

Once you have completed a pilot program, assess its success using the measures that have been established. Working with your sponsors and critical constituents, decide if you would like to expand the program, try a different project or scrap it.

If you decide to expand the program, begin to build the infrastructure for scaling the operation. Inserting telemedicine into the organization involves establishing billing guidelines. (See Chapter 10)

Collaborating with the risk, legal and regulatory teams is important (see Chapter 12) since they will help to ensure compliance, as well as protecting the organization from privacy leaks. This group can often assist with policy writing, as well.

Establishing an IT infrastructure including technology standards and data storage and transfer requirements is vital so that the telemedicine program projects seamlessly exchange data. Addressing the data transfers between EHRs and health information exchanges (HIEs) is also essential.

Lastly, ensure clinical and operational workflow guidelines closely integrate the existing operations with the new telemedicine services. Staffing should be scheduled, and all applicable staff, adequately trained in the operating procedures, as well as the consenting, data flows, and technology support services.

Chapter 9

Developing a Business Case

Before the pandemic, developing a business case for telemedicine was complicated. There were few direct revenue generation examples (although some!) The pandemic has fundamentally changed the telemedicine business case. CMS billing guidelines now offer direct compensation for telemedicine visits as though they are in-person visits. While some of these changes may be temporary, many have already been made permanent. Telemedicine is not simply a revenue-generating tool. Sometimes its most important value propositions do not generate revenue. Below are viable financial models associated with telehealth. They include:

Direct Revenue Generation

CMS has changed many of the arcane and difficult telemedicine billing requirements, allowing many more telemedicine "visits" to be billed as though they are in-person encounters. And private insurers have followed the CMS lead.

There are also other ways to use telemedicine to expand opportunities to generate revenue. For example, healthcare providers can offer specialist services to rural entities. They can expand their services beyond their geography. They can extend services into prisons, schools, communities, and individuals. Special services like genetic counseling, fertility counseling, opioid treatment, sexual health, and others provide opportunities for healthcare professionals to add revenue streams and new patients to their practice.

Cost Avoidance for "Capitated or At-Risk" Patients

When an organization is "at-risk" for the overall cost of care associated with a population's health, the patient must use the most cost-effective approach to seek care. Therefore, redirecting an allergy-suffering patient from the emergency department on the weekends to a telemedicine option with distant providers would significantly save the patient and the hospital.

Cost Reduction

Physicians, and especially specialists, are an expensive resource. The use of telemedicine extends these precious resources to additional hospitals by relieving physicians from unnecessary travel. It also offers the physician at home to see home-bound or skilled nursing patients as needed instead of unnecessary trips to facilities.

Reduce Length of Stay in the Acute Setting

Hospitalized patients spend most of their time waiting to see physicians to be examined or for tests to be ordered. Telemedicine can bring the physicians to the bedside more swiftly so that tests can be ordered and results reviewed. There is the potential for the length of stay to be reduced. In addition, continuous monitoring of patients in the intensive care unit and neonatal units has reduced the length of hospitalization and provided patients with additional care coverage.

Reduce Readmissions

Monitoring patients at home or in a skilled nursing facility, especially those patients with complex chronic conditions, can reduce readmissions. Patients and facilities are less likely to arrive back in the emergency department to see a physician "just in case it's serious."

New Business Models

There are many areas in healthcare where people are willing to pay cash for consultations, for example, fertility consultations, genetic consulting, and plastic surgery consultations. A viable, revenue-generating telemedicine business can be created worldwide if people are willing to pay for the encounter. Specialists with excellent reputations can develop another revenue source using telemedicine.

Second Opinion Services

Johns Hopkins and Barrow Brain and Spine are using telemedicine to offer second opinions. Patients send their scans, medical records, and physician opinions to specialists skilled at assessing specific conditions. If the physicians believe they can assist the patient, they contact the patient and offer their services. It is a way for a powerful organization to extend its brand and for patients to consult with prominent specialists.

Examples of Telemedicine Uses

Type of Telemedicine service	Type of telemedicine service	Setting	Synchronous /Asynchronous	Value proposition
ICU / NICU monitoring	Continuous Monitoring or Provider to Consumer	Acute	S	Anticipate adverse events, higher level of care, reduction in lengths of stay, patient satisfaction
Telestroke Networks, Behavioral Health	Provider to provider to consumer	Acute, Ambulatory	S	Balance workforce, provide specialists to rural areas
Dermatology, Pathology	Provider to provider	Acute or Ambulatory	A	Convenience
Internal medicine doctor discusses case with cardiologist	Provider to provider consults	Acute or Ambulatory	S	Medical Home Model, better quality of care, supports continuum of care

Tumor Boards, Grand Rounds, Project Echo	Medical Education	Acute or Ambulatory	S, A	Knowledge transfer, professional education
Chronic Complex patient visits	Provider to existing patient	Ambulatory	S	Patient convenience, closer monitoring of care
Various companies including Teladoc, American Well, Doctor on Demand	Provider to new patient (on demand)	Ambulatory, Occupational Health	S	Cost avoidance
Post-Discharge CHF patients monitored	Home monitoring	Ambulatory	S	Cost avoidance, pop health management
Radiology images read by radiologists	Image Sharing	Acute and Ambulatory	A	Revenue Generation

Chapter 10

Is Your Telemedicine Encounter Billable?

Before COVID, billing telemedicine encounters was complicated. As previously mentioned, there were significant changes made during the pandemic. Below is the text from the CMS fact sheet:

- *Effective for services starting March 6, 2020 and for the duration of the COVID-19 Public Health Emergency,* ***Medicare will make payment for Medicare telehealth services furnished to patients in broader circumstances.***
- ***These visits are considered the same as in-person visits and are paid at the same rate as regular, in-person visits.***
- *Starting March 6, 2020 and for the duration of the COVID-19 Public Health Emergency,* ***Medicare will make payment for professional services furnished to***

beneficiaries in all areas of the country in all settings.

- *While they must generally travel to or be located in certain types of originating sites such as a physician's office, skilled nursing facility or hospital for the visit, effective for services starting March 6, 2020 and for the duration of the COVID-19 Public Health Emergency, Medicare will make payment for Medicare telehealth services furnished to beneficiaries in any healthcare facility and in their home.*
- *The Medicare coinsurance and deductible would generally apply to these services. However, the HHS Office of Inspector General (OIG) is providing flexibility for healthcare providers to reduce or waive cost-sharing for telehealth visits paid by federal healthcare programs.*
- *To the extent the 1135 waiver requires an established relationship, HHS will not conduct audits to ensure that such a prior relationship existed for claims submitted during this public health emergency.*

https://www.cms.gov/newsroom/fact-sheets/medicare-telemedicine-health-care-provider-fact-sheet

TYPE OF SERVICE	WHAT IS THE SERVICE?	HCPCS/CPT CODE	Patient Relationship with Provider
MEDICARE TELEHEALTH VISITS	A visit with a provider that uses telecommunication systems between a provider and a patient.	Common telehealth services include: • 99201-99215 (Office or other outpatient visits) • G0425-G0427 (Telehealth consultations, emergency department or initial inpatient) • G0406-G0408 (Follow-up inpatient telehealth consultations furnished to beneficiaries in hospitals or SNFs) For a complete list: https://www.cms.gov/Medicare/Medicare-General-Information/Telehealth/Telehealth-Codes	For new* or established patients. *To the extent the 1135 waiver requires an established relationship. HHS will not conduct audits to ensure that such a prior relationship existed for claims submitted during this public health emergency
VIRTUAL CHECK-IN	A brief (5-10 minutes) check in with your practitioner via telephone or other telecommunications device to decide whether an office visit or other service is needed. A remote evaluation of recorded video and/or images submitted by an established patient.	• HCPCS code G2012 • HCPCS code G2010	For established patients.
E-VISITS	A communication between a patient and their provider through an online patient portal.	• 99421 • 99422 • 99423 • G2061 • G2062 • G2063	For established patients.

Previously, the reimbursement for telehealth services has been complex. It depended on the payer source, the type of telehealth interaction, patient geography, special coding, and a host of other dependencies.

Each payer source, Medicare, Medicaid, and Private Payers, had different definitions and parameters for billing. They delineated and defined key elements associated with billing guidelines. Referring to their guiding policy was critical to determining their unique criteria. Sometimes, it was a challenge to find the most current policy. For example, Medicare had eight different source documents that guide telehealth billing. Post-pandemic, it is unclear whether the simplicity of the CMS fact sheet listed above will prevail or if there will be a return to the previously complex approach.

Because it is unclear what will happen after the pandemic, the previous billing requirements are listed below.

PAST BILLING MODEL:

Assisted providers used these steps to assess whether or not the telemedicine encounter was billable. These criteria may return in some form. This is only a guide. Check with your private payer, Medicare or Medicaid technical expert, and organization billing staff to verify!

1. Identify the Payer

It will likely be Medicare, Medicaid, or a private payer. There are many permutations, including the Medicare

Advantage payers, the accountable care organizations, health maintenance organizations, etc., but for simple demonstration purposes, assume there are only three buckets.

2. Determine the Five Factors Associated with Reimbursement, including:

a. What is the type of telehealth transaction?

Synchronous: If the transaction is synchronous or occurring simultaneously, like a video conferencing application, it is quite possibly billable. Synchronous interactions require webcam use.

Asynchronous: If the transaction is a scan, photo, or some other type of static document captured and then sent to a provider for review later, it is considered an "asynchronous" or "Store and Forward" telemedicine transaction. There are a few states, namely Alaska and Hawaii, where Medicare will reimburse for these expenses. Nevertheless, for the most part, they are unbillable.

Monitoring: Remote monitoring is billable as a remote or ambulatory service with code 99490. It is not yet billable in the acute environment.

b. Is there a geographic or rural requirement?

Most payers apply a geographic restriction or definition to the telemedicine encounter in order to allow billing for services. Medicare defines as "rural" as a non-metropolitan Statistical Area or Health Professional Shortage Area

c.Where is the telemedicine encounter initiated or "Site-type?"

Qualified site types vary depending upon the payer. For Medicare, the qualified sites to initiate or receive billable telemedicine encounters are Physician or provider offices, Hospitals, Critical Access Hospitals, Rural Health Clinics, Federally Qualified Health Centers, Hospital-based or CAH-based Renal Dialysis Centers (including satellites), Skilled Nursing Facilities (SNF), and Community Mental Health Centers.

d.Who is the practitioner, and are they deemed eligible?

The eligible practitioner type also varies depending upon the payer. For Medicare, the eligible practitioners allowed to bill for telemedicine encounters are Physicians, Nurse Practitioners, Physician Assistants, Nurse Midwives, Clinical Nurse Specialists (CNS), Clinical Psychologists, and Clinical Social Workers.

e.Does the coding accurately reflect the telemedicine encounter?

When submitting a bill to Medicare, Medicaid, or Private Payers, the coding should be similar to a non-telemedicine encounter. The difference is the coding. Coders should add GT or GQ modifiers to the code number. Some providers choose not to do so, but this practice runs the risk of audit irregularities that could result in fines.

Remote patient monitoring is different. There are specific different codes that can be billed for remote patient monitoring, but it is an ever-evolving area of CMS guidance, so check out CMS. 99490 and additional codes can be your friend!

f. State by State variations

Varying from state to state, other aspects affect the telemedicine encounter, including whether or not a telemedicine coordinator is present and if a physician relationship was established by an in-person encounter.

PREVIOUS BILLING REQUIREMENTS (PRE-PANDEMIC) including because this chart may be used in the future, post-pandemic.

Key element	Medicare	Medicaid*	Private Payers
Definition of telehealth	An **interactive audio and video** telecommunications system must be used that permits **real-time communication** between you, at the distant site, and the beneficiary, at the originating site. **Asynchronous "store and forward"** technology is **not permitted** (except for demonstration programs.)	Different states vary. For example, in Arizona, both asynchronous and synchronous services are billable.	Nearly every private payer uses Medicare's definition or a very similar one.
Rural designation required by originating site?	Yes	Varies	Varies
Rural Definition	HPSA, non-MSA, Rural census tract as determined by Office of Rural Health Policy within HRSA (website available for determination: http://datawarehouse.hrsa.gov/ telehealthAdvisor/telehe	Varies	Varies

	althEligibility.aspx		
Eligible originating facility site	1. Physician or provider office 2. Hospitals 3. Critical Access Hospitals 4. Rural Health Clinics 5. Federally Qualified Health Centers 6. Hospital-based or CAH-based Renal Dialysis Centers (including satellites) 7. Skilled Nursing Facilities (SNF); 8. Community Mental Health Centers	Varies by State: As an example, AZ includes: *1. IHS clinic* *2. Tribally-governed 638 facility* *3. Urban clinic for Native Americans* *4. Office of a physician or other practitioner* *5. Hospital* *6. Federally qualified health center (FQHC)*	Nearly every private payer uses Medicare's definition or a very similar one.
Eligible distant site practitioners	1. Physicians 2. Nurse Practitioners 3. Physician Assistants 4. Nurse-Midwives 5. Clinical nurse specialists (CNS) 6. Clinical psychologists and clinical social workers	Varies	Often, providers are members of their network.

Covered Specialties	See Rural health Fact Sheer Series (ICM 901705, April 2014)	Varies	Varies but is often more restrictive than Medicare.
Other	1. Distant sites are paid the provider fee. 2. Originating sites are paid an originating site facility fee ONLY (HCPCS Code Q3014.)	Varies but often does NOT pay an originating site fee	Unknown

Chapter 11

Technology and data integration

Even pre-pandemic, there have been significant consolidation and dynamic changes in the telemedicine industry. From an industry with quite a few small players and just one or two large ones (Teladoc, InTouch), the industry consolidation has resulted in about four to five prominent players (American Well, Teladoc, Doctor on Demand, and lesser smaller ones. Recently, Walmart purchased MeMD. American Well purchased Avizia. Teladoc merged with Livongo and purchased InTouch. Philips acquired BioTelemetry. And, insurance companies are also buying telemedicine companies, as per the recent acquisition by BlueCross/Blue Shield of MDLive. Large electronic health record (EHR) technology vendors are also working to integrate telemedicine into their platforms. Of course, the dynamic nature of technology and industry means this will change. And, several prominent players like Amazon are signaling they will enter the telemedicine/healthcare field, meaning further disruption is likely.

Because these large companies have active sales forces, technology vendors often drive telemedicine projects. It is vital to create a needs analysis of your practice or hospital's telemedicine requirements before selecting the technology. That said, at some point, technology must be selected to support the program's operations. Technology is critical to ensuring a successful launch and ultimately affects your ability to scale the program.

Choosing a technology vendor should be initiated with a survey of applicable vendors. Usually, sending a request for information (RFI) to many vendors will serve that purpose. After reviewing the RFI responses, select the top four vendors to send a Request for Proposal (RFP) with all of the detailed questions required by the sponsors and constituents previously identified. Using a score sheet and checking references keeps the process logical, fair, and thorough.

Software Options

The software can range dramatically from custom solutions, proprietary systems, or HIPAA-compliant video technology. Below is a partial but certainly not exhaustive list of potential vendors in each space.

Type of Program	Care Setting 1	Care Setting 2	Potential Technology Vendors
Intensive Care Unit Monitoring	Hospital	NA	**Philips, Hicuity Health**
Telestroke	Hospital	Community Hospital	**InTouch Health (part of Teladoc), Specialists on Call**
Telepsychiatry	Hospital	Clinic	**VSee, eVisit, InTouch Health, American Well, Zoom**

Teleurgent Care	Clinic	Home	Wide range including American Well, **Doctor on Demand, American Well, Teladoc, Zoom**
General Practice Support	Clinic	Home	**Mend.com, Doxy.me, AMCHealth** VSee, Teladoc

Hardware Device options

Various hardware solutions can be used to enable telemedicine encounters. For this section, we are not covering intensive care monitoring.

Telemedicine Carts

A medical-grade telemedicine cart can be purchased for several thousand dollars for specialized care that requires precision and cleanliness. A cart enables peripherals to be added that can enhance the examination. Telemedicine cart strengths as a tool include medical-grade quality, ability to be cleaned, security, and additional peripherals tools to enhance examinations, like otoscopes, stethoscopes, and heart monitors. Telemedicine cart disadvantages are cost, floor space, and storage. Two leading telemedicine cart vendors are American Well and Global Med.

Tablet With or Without a Stand

Tablets can be purchased for hundreds of dollars, making them an affordable solution, especially for the skilled nursing or home setting. Tablet advantages are that it is inexpensive, requires little training, and is portable. The tablet's disadvantages are that it can be challenging to locate, easily "borrowed," difficult to clean, and offers few medical-grade peripherals.

Laptop Computer with Web or Video Camera

A simple laptop computer with a web or video camera can be used to power telemedicine. Acquiring a computer costs more than a tablet but significantly less than a telemedicine cart. The advantages of a laptop computer are that it is inexpensive and people already know how to use it. The disadvantages are that the computer can "walk away," is difficult to clean, and offers few medical-grade peripherals.

Data Integration

Telemedicine is unlikely to become integrated into the core operations of an organization until the data can easily flow to and from existing data sources. Every organization's data is handled differently. Some have a health information exchange, others have a proprietary data mart, and others have large data warehouses. Telemedicine encounters should be integrated into the electronic health record. Avoid the temptation to store the data in a "one-off" location. Some EHR software companies are incorporating telemedicine into their platform.

Tap into the expertise of your technology teams. They will appreciate your questions about data formatting. As you identify the data and its flow, members of the data team can offer guidance about the HL7 or Consolidated Clinical Document Architecture (CCDA) standards. They will help you create a data plan.

Include the data scientists, communication experts, and network engineers in the telemedicine project. They add value and offer a broad perspective.

Chapter 12

Telemedicine Staffing

As telemedicine grows, professionals need to create, run, and work within the telemedicine programs. There is little agreement about how to "rank" or name telemedicine program positions. Job titles include telehealth coordinator, telemedicine program director, telemedicine program manager, and telehealth senior manager, to name a few. One study showed nearly 30 different titles for roughly the same job. Below are typical jobs associated with telemedicine programs. Because the field is not yet mature, programs are staffed with people entering from other fields. Consequently, each category includes a descriptor and important skills professionals may wish to acquire should they want to be considered for roles in successful telemedicine programs.

Clinical

Clinical positions include nurses, physicians, nurse practitioners, and physician assistants. Increasingly, some programs, like the continuous monitoring programs, are using nursing assistants or medical technicians. If you are currently a clinician and would like to work in the field, look for opportunities to participate in pilot programs or introduce telemedicine into your organization. Across the country, there are excellent certificate and degree programs emphasizing clinical informatics.

The key to embarking upon telemedicine as a clinician is to show an interest in the field. Read about it. Subscribe to the mailing lists detailed in the appendix. In addition, learn about technology. Often, nurses and physicians understand some core medical systems but may not be as facile with different types of technology. Learn how to use the various workstations on wheels, iPads, computers, and electronic medical records. If you are a physician, there are services you can register to appear as an on-call physician. You can experiment with different services with little commitment, except to show up to your shift, especially in the low acuity urgent care space. If you are a psychiatrist or psychologist, some services will welcome you. Some of the services to investigate include Doctor on Demand, Teladoc, American Well, and others.

Technology

Sometimes telemedicine programs rest in the information technology (IT) department. This practice is not advisable, as the mission of most IT departments in healthcare organizations is to keep the organization secure. Developing innovative projects and programs that open the organization to new technologies, processes, and data directly opposes the mission. By its very nature, healthcare innovation, including telemedicine, challenges the status quo. That said, telemedicine programs will likely encounter the IT department at some point, even if they are not located in that department.

Telemedicine positions in the IT department are program manager positions, data engineering positions, and telemedicine coordinator positions. If you are located in the IT department and wish to embark upon telemedicine, begin to learn about it, sit on the technology selection committee, and understand the interaction between IT and the clinical team using telemedicine. There is a strong need for people to understand BOTH the clinical aspects of telemedicine and the technology required to operate it. Ideally, once both aspects are understood, a valuable professional would effectively communicate the concepts and serve as a liaison between the disparate teams.

Project Management

All telemedicine projects require project management. Learning the key project management principles and then applying them to telemedicine projects is another way to enter the field. Telemedicine projects can be approached like other information technology projects. They are complex projects with multiple elements and a variety of stakeholders.

Program Management

Most telemedicine programs require a person who understands all aspects of the telemedicine proposition. Program management requires an understanding of the financial, legal, technological, and clinical aspects of telemedicine. It does not require a clinical degree, but often, program managers are nurses who have obtained additional training in project management, informatics, or technology.

Administration

An operations executive who is assigned that task by senior leadership initiates some telemedicine programs. Once the program is activated, the program adds personnel, like program managers, clinicians, and technologists. Healthcare executives and administrators assigned this role are uniquely positioned to build a career in telemedicine and run even larger telemedicine operations. Whether or not an administrator is appointed a formal role, it is important to identify an administrator to help champion the project. Both a physician leader and an administrator/leader as sponsors will facilitate program success.

Chapter 13

Other Operational Considerations

Training

Training for the clinicians that will be conducting telemedicine encounters is critical. The training should include not just the physicians but also the scribes, medical assistants, nurses, and other personnel that will be "touching" the system. The physician may be on the screen but getting the system set up and positioned correctly requires other personnel. Encourage the program manager/non-clinician to conduct hands-on training in the setting where telemedicine will be performed. All too often, there is a gap between the project plan and clinical realities. Working side by side with clinicians will allow the program/project manager the opportunity to identify the training gaps or (sometimes low-tech) clinical aids to encourage the adoption of the new technologies.

Communications

As a best practice, all stakeholders affected by the telemedicine project should be apprised of the project. Patients, the quality team, administrators, leaders, nurses, and staff may all be impacted. Having a consistent and concise message about the vision, impact, benefits, and operational details is critical to project success. As is critical for any change management project, identifying the key stakeholders, influencers, nay-sayers, and resisters and tailoring the communications to them will ease the path to adoption.

Risk

Every healthcare organization has a risk management department. Conferring with that team is advisable in the event that there are precautions that must be taken to reduce any potential negative impact. Although there have been very few legal challenges and lawsuits pertaining to telemedicine care, it's only a matter of time before it happens. Working with physicians, practice administrators, and hospital executives to ensure they are covered by the malpractice coverage and other risk-management tools is advisable. The American Society for Health Care Risk Management has an excellent whitepaper addressing telemedicine risk.

Workflows

Creating a flow chart of the telemedicine encounter is a valuable tool to share with staff. It gives everyone an overview of the entire process and allows him or her to digest and comment on the operational steps. Presenting the workflows during training gives staff the opportunity to identify any items that may have been missed in the workflow development.

Printed Guides or Job Aids

Creating a paper job aid that can sit with the equipment or in the pocket of a provider is a valuable tool for providers and staff. Until the telemedicine processes and methods become incorporated into their everyday job tasks, there is a learning curve.

Having a printed job aid or guide supports the new processes and supports the change management goals.

Part 4 Laws, Regulations, and Policy

Chapter 14

Laws and Regulations

Perhaps the most complex issues associated with telehealth are the legal issues. A thorough understanding of the legal and regulatory issues related to telehealth is critical to successful deployment. Again, the pandemic changed some of the laws and regulations associated with telemedicine adoption and use.

The US Federal government, realizing the quick adoption of telemedicine would require some legal, safe harbors, created a few of them. The Stark Law and Anti-Kickback Statute were revised with a final OIG ruling to support value-based arrangements, patient engagement, care coordination, and cybersecurity. The Final Rule not only created six new safe harbors but modified five existing sale harbors. According to one attorney, "the changes to the Anti-Kickback regulations are good news for digital health innovation and the shift to value-based care." Specifically, "These new protections allow players in the digital health space – including Remote Patient Monitoring companies, telehealth companies, and healthcare predictive analytics platforms – to take on an unprecedented role in helping healthcare providers move the needle on patient outcomes and costs by providing in-kind and even monetary remuneration to these providers in the form of free or reduced-cost items/services or shared savings arrangements."

Below are common issues and resources important to address as you grow telemedicine within your organization. NOTE: The author is not an attorney. This information should be used for guidance and research purposes only. Seek professional legal services by licensed professionals.

Malpractice Insurance

Organizations should understand and review the physician or provider malpractice limits and requirements of their coverage pertaining to telemedicine. If a telemedicine program includes patient visits in non-specified locations, there is a potential for malpractice coverage being inapplicable.

Without licensure in the patient's location (State or Country), the physician or provider risks practicing medicine without a license. Most professional liability insurance policies specifically exclude coverage for unlicensed activities; some states require professional liability underwriters to cover practice that extends beyond state borders, and some do not.

Privacy of Patient Data and Health Information

Address the organization's expectations around the applicable federal and state legal requirements of medical/health information privacy, including compliance with the Health Insurance Portability and Accountability Act (HIPAA) and state privacy, confidentiality, security, and medical retention rules. Some organizations refer physicians to "Standards for Privacy of Individually Identifiable Health Information," issued by the Department of Health and Human Services (HHS).

Jurisdiction

Because laws vary from state to state, organizations should specify the policies' ruling jurisdiction. Most policies are subject to a particular state's laws, statutes, and regulations, the Centers for Medicaid and Medicare, and any other applicable or overriding legal entities. You may want to add a disclaimer due to telemedicine's fluid and changing nature, the most current laws, statutes, and regulations apply.

Licensure

Prior to the pandemic, the location of the patient when the telemedicine encounter occurs is the determining factor for physician or provider licensure. In other words, the practice of telemedicine occurs where the patient is located when the telemedicine technologies are used. Therefore, a physician or provider must be licensed by, or be under the jurisdiction of, the medical board of the state where the patient is located. Physicians or providers who treat or prescribe via telemedicine are practicing medicine and must possess appropriate licensure in all jurisdictions where patients receive care. HRSA provided a comprehensive review of licensure with specific attention paid to telehealth with its Senate report 111-66.

However, the emergent nature of COVID forced some requirements to be modified. Forty-one states, Guam, US Virgin Islands, Puerto Rico, Northern Mariana Islands, Washington DC, have altered the licensing requirements for telehealth in response to COVID-19. The modifications include: allowing a telephone without video to "count" as a telemedicine visit, special purpose licensure for physicians, waiver of physician licensure in the state, dropping the requirement for preexisting provider-patient relationships, temporary licensure in other states, relaxation of privacy laws related to audio and video telehealth appointments, and more. The state-by-state guide published by the Federation of State Medical Boards can be accessed here.

Chapter 15

Interstate Licensure Compact

Telehealth services require that the physician be licensed in the state where the patient is physically located. Because each state licenses its physicians, and besides the veteran's administration, there is no federal mechanism to license physicians, the question of license portability is being investigated. A medical licensure compact for physicians is in process. A nursing compact already exists.

Telemedicine currently requires physicians to become licensed in each state where they are practicing medicine. Technology is changing the definition of an "exam." It is enabling physicians to examine, diagnose, and treat a patient without regard to geography. Physicians wishing to practice in multiple states must become licensed in each state where patients may reside. Multi-state licensure, therefore, becomes expensive and burdensome for physicians practicing telemedicine.

Nurses can use their licenses across states via reciprocity and a multi-state compact that eases the burden of licensure and enhances license portability.

In 2013, a number of state medical boards, the Federation of State Medical Boards, and experts from the Council of State Governments, and interested stakeholder groups began to explore forming an interstate compact for physicians. Eighteen months later, a compact was drafted that is being contemplated by physicians, state medical boards, and state legislatures.

"An interstate compact is a legal agreement among participating states that allows them to work closely together to address issues of mutual concern that cross state borders. Hundreds of compacts exist in the United States, and they have helped states address everything from shared water use to transportation issues.

In the case of the Interstate Medical Licensure Compact, it is an agreement that allows states to work together to significantly streamline the licensing process for physicians who want to practice in multiple states."

Below are the eight consensus principles quoted directly from the FSMB website. They include:

•Participation in an interstate compact for medical licensure will be strictly voluntary for both physicians and state boards of medicine.

•Participation in an interstate compact creates another pathway for licensure but does not otherwise change a state's existing Medical Practice Act.

•The practice of medicine occurs where the patient is located at the time of the physician-patient encounter. Therefore, it requires the physician to be under the jurisdiction of the state medical board where the patient is located.

•An interstate compact for medical licensure will establish a mechanism whereby any physician practicing in the state will be known by and under the state medical board's jurisdiction where the practice occurs.

•Regulatory authority will remain with the participating state medical boards and will not be delegated to any entity that would administer a compact.

•A physician practicing under an interstate compact is bound to comply with each compact state's statutes, rules, and regulations wherein he/she chooses to practice.

•State boards participating in an interstate compact must share complaint / investigative information.

•The license to practice can be revoked by any or all of the compact states.

State legislatures and medical boards are currently considering draft legislation to participate in the Interstate Medical Licensure Compact. To date, 30 states, the District of Columbia and Guam, have joined the compact.

Author's note: The progress towards the Interstate Medical Licensure Compact seems to have stalled (perhaps due to the pandemic and relaxing of licensure rules.) Monitor the FSMB and IMLC website for updates when the post-pandemic world changes the shape of telemedicine and multistate licensure.

Chapter 16

Policy

It is beneficial for healthcare organizations to create telemedicine policies that are consistent and aligned with existing in-person clinical care policies. New policies to address telemedicine use during the pandemic are advisable. After the special pandemic rules are lifted, the policies will need to be revised again to be consistent with the law, rules, and regulatory environment.

Before the pandemic, I advised, if telemedicine is treated as a "one-off" or unique program, the likelihood of it growing to the enterprise level is very low. Policies guide establishing professional medical practices while using telemedicine technologies. They define the standards of care and interactions both in delivering medical services directly to patients and between clinicians while using telemedicine technologies.

Delineating clinical, documentation, and quality standards will increase the likelihood of sustaining successful telemedicine encounters. The use of technology can wedge a gap between patient and provider. As such, it is important in policy to encourage providers to use communication tools and approaches that bridge the natural gap that occurs during the use of technology.

While writing policies about telemedicine, it is important to define the types of telemedicine that are included and those that are excluded. For example, telemedicine policies may include or exclude audio-only telephony, routine e-mail, instant messaging, and fax. Define the terms of telemedicine so that it addresses synchronous, asynchronous, and continuous monitoring. Important elements of policies may include:

Consent

Many hospitals or providers have incorporated telemedicine into their general consent forms, but if your organization has not, it is worth considering a consent form presented to the patient at the time of the telemedicine encounter.

Physicians and Prescribing

When pharmaceuticals are prescribed during the telemedicine encounter, policies that address patient safety in the absence of a traditional physical examination are advisable. Policies should include measures to guarantee the identity of the patient, establish a patient/provider relationship, and create detailed documentation for the clinical evaluation and resulting prescription. Record retention policies should reflect organizational standards. Note: It is illegal to prescribe controlled substances using telemedicine.

Policies should delineate that physicians or providers should not establish or maintain preferred relationships with any pharmacy. There should not be an exchange of consideration, benefit, or any type of remuneration for transmitting prescriptions to or recommending a pharmacy.

Credentialing

Hospitals sometimes require that physicians and providers performing telemedicine services be credentialed according to the medical staff by-laws, policies, and procedures. In particular, credentialing is an essential consideration for hospital-based telemedicine activities. Some hospitals offer expedited and abbreviated credentialing if the physician will not see patients on the hospital premises. Consult with the medical staff services to develop policies that are consistent with the organization's existing policies.

Privileging

Some hospitals require that any physician/provider providing telemedicine services on their behalf apply for and maintain privileges according to their employing or contracting entity's processes and standards. They will often reference the medical staff bylaws, policies, and procedures, as well as Medicare requirements.

Documentation

A telemedicine encounter is a medical encounter. If a patient medical record already exists, it is essential to document the encounter. If there is no pre-existing patient record, it is recommended that a medical record be created for all telemedicine patients, whether or not one already exists. The record should specify that the visit has occurred via telemedicine.

Final thoughts

Telemedicine is the present and future of medicine. After years of languishing, finally, the pandemic has pushed it to adoption levels never before experienced. The laws have been changed, CMS has addressed billing (the highest hurdle) and lowered technology barriers. People who never before "saw" a doctor through their phones or computer have done it. Or they are aware the option exists. By some estimates, post-COVID-19, telemedicine will be a $250 Billion industry. The willingness of patients to use telemedicine, favorable consumer perception, investment, regulatory changes, convenience, and the general integration of technology in all aspects of our lives, point to enduring telemedicine use.

As the pandemic subsides and our post-pandemic world is established, telemedicine will continue to morph and change. Lawsuits related to telemedicine could complicate the eventual adoption, as could CMS's reversal of billing or regulatory changes.

One thing is clear; telemedicine continues to have enormous growth potential. Adopting its use into hospitals, long-term care facilities, private practices, schools, prisons, and even ambulances will change and improve healthcare. It can reach rural, low-income, indigenous peoples, and elderly patients who may have postponed care due to location or unfamiliarity with technology.

Although telemedicine programs during the pandemic have been stood up quickly, they deserve the same rigor and quality-based scrutiny associated with in-person care. Developing a comprehensive program infrastructure similar to that associated with traditional care will increase the likelihood of enterprise adoption and growth. Although implementing telemedicine is complex and challenging, it is well worth bringing care to patients who need a different type of healthcare setting.

Telemedicine is a valuable tool as healthcare professionals work to achieve the "Triple Aim" of better healthcare, lower costs, and improved population health. As technology improves, telemedicine will incorporate virtual reality, augmented reality, predictive data analytics, and improved technology. Anywhere someone has access to the internet, a person will have access to medical care.

APPENDIX

Organizations to Join

- American Telemedicine Association: https://www.americantelemed.org
- HIMSS: Health Information and Management Systems Society- http://www.himss.org
- AHIMA: American Health Information Management Association- https://www.ahima.org
- cTel: Center for Telehealth and e-Health Law: https://www.ctel-innovations.com
- National Technology Center – Telehealth Technology Assessment Resource Center: https://telehealthtechnology.org/

Regional Telehealth Centers are a system of telehealth regional resource centers assisting rural entities. They offer excellent resources. They do not provide funding but provide technical assistance, consulting, and matchmaking between physicians, vendors, and health organizations.

Find your resource center at the map at https://www.telehealthresourcecenter.org

- Northwest Regional Telehealth Resource Center: https://www.nrtrc.org
- California Telehealth Resource Center: https://www.caltrc.org
- Southwest Telehealth Resource Center: https://www.southwesttrc.org
- Great Plains Telehealth Resource and Assistance Center: https://www.gptrac.org
- Heartland Telehealth Resource Center: https://www.heartlandtrc.org
- TEXLA Telehealth Resource Center: https://www.texlatrc.org
- Northeast Telehealth Resource Center: https://www.netrc.org
- Upper Midwest Telehealth Resource Center: https://www.umtrc.org
- MidAtlantic Telehealth Resource Center: https://www.matrc.org
- South Central Telehealth Resource Center: https://www.learntelehealth.org

- Southeast Telehealth Resource Center: https://www.gatelehealth.org
- Pacific Basin Telehealth Resource Center: https://www.pbtrc.org

Subscribe to these Mailing Lists

- Center for Connected Health Policy: http://www.cchpca.org
- cTel: http://ctel-innovations.com/
- Federal Telemedicine News: https://www.federaltelemedicine.com
- Gartner: https://www.gartner.com
- Health Affairs: https://www.healthaffairs.org
- Healthcare Dive: https://www.healthcaredive.com
- Healthcare Law Today: https://www.healthcarelawtoday.com
- National Academy Press: https://www.nap.edu
- ONC Health IT: https://www.healthit.gov
- Rock Weekly: https://rockhealth.com/rock-weekly/

- mHealth Intelligence: https://www.mhealthintelligence.com
- Connected Health Pulse: https://www.connectedhealthpulse.com/
- HealthcareIT News: https://www.healthcareitnews.com/
- MobiHealthNews: https://www.mobihealthnews.com/
- Healthcare Innovation: https://www.hcinnovationgroup.com/
- Wheel: https://www.wheel.com/blog
- Fierce IT: https://fiercehealthcare.com/it
- Healio: https://www.healio.com

Resource Links

Billing

- Eligibility link at HRSA: https://data.hrsa.gov/tools/medicare/telehealth
- Link to CMS ruling: http://www.cms.gov

Accreditation

- URAC: https://www.urac.org/accreditation-cert/telehealth-accreditation/
- The Joint Commission: https://www.jointcommission.org

Policy and Legislation

- Telehealth Medicaid and State Policy and Interactive Map: https://www.cchpca.org/resources/state-telehealth-laws-and-reimbursement-policies-report-spring-2021/
- State Telemedicine Gaps Report:

https://www.americantelemed.org/initiatives/2019-state-of-the-states-report-coverage-and-reimbursement/

- Privacy and policy documents at the HHS Office for Civil Rights Web site: www.hhs.gov/ocr/hipaa

Legal Resources

- A 50-State Survey of Telehealth legalities is found at the American Health Lawyers Association (AHLA) site. https://www.americanhealthlaw.org/
  The publication is at: https://educate.americanhealthlaw.org/local/catalog/view/product.php?productid=458 (This is the 2017, 2nd edition. It will not address COVID changes but still provides an excellent summary.)

- Epstein Becker Green Telemental/Telebehavioral Health 50-state Survey: https://e-coms.ebglaw.com/61/260/landing-pages/thank-you---accept.asp

- State Laws and Reimbursement Policies: The Center for Connected Health has an excellent dropdown menu sorting their resources by topic, federal laws, and each state's laws and regulations associated with telemedicine. https://www.cchpca.org/

- Licensure gap analysis: A 50-state gap analysis associated with physician practice standards and licensure is found at the American Telemedicine Association site. It was published in 2017, so it may be out of date. https://utn.org/resources/downloads/50-state-telemedicine-gaps-analysis-physician-practice-standards-licensure.pdf

- Credentialing and Privileging: Credentialing and privileging is a challenging issue for telehealth practitioners and the organizations that wish to use them. CMS issued a final rule in July 2011. However, since then, there was a Joint Commission standard regarding telemedicine revisions. (See below.) http://www.gpo.gov/fdsys/pkg/FR-2011-05-05/pdf/2011-10875.pdf https://www.jointcommission.org/-/media/tjc/documents/standards/jc-requirements/revisions_telemedicine_standardspdf.pdf?db=web&hash=80DD5BCB3FE622C42BEE956C35611376

Trends to Watch

Medicare Billing:

https://www.cms.gov/medicare/medicare-general-information/telehealth/

Interstate licensure Compact:

https://www.imlcc.org

Federation of State Medical Boards (Compact):

https://www.fsmb.org/Media/Default/PDF/Advocacy/Interstate%20Medical%20Licensure%20Compact%20(FINAL).pdf

Additional resources and links referenced in the text related to COVID-19:

Centers for Disease Control/Telemedicine Trends:

https://www.cdc.gov/mmwr/volumes/69/wr/mm6943a3.htm

https://www.cdc.gov/mmwr/volumes/70/wr/mm7007a3.htm

American Medical Association and McKinsey and Co. / Post COVID Telemedicine Opportunity:

https://www.ama-assn.org/practice-management/digital/after-covid-19-250-billion-care-could-shift-telehealth

https://www.mckinsey.com/industries/healthcare-systems-and-services/our-insights/telehealth-a-quarter-trillion-dollar-post-covid-19-reality#

Telemedicine Use During COVID

https://www.ncbi.nlm.nih.gov/pmc/articles/PMC7395209/

https://www.hhs.gov/coronavirus/telehealth/index.html

https://www.healio.com/news/primary-care/20210201/telehealth-used-in-301-of-visits-during-covid19-pandemic

https://www.kff.org/medicare/issue-brief/medicare-and-telehealth-coverage-and-use-during-the-covid-19-pandemic-and-options-for-the-future/

https://www.ama-assn.org/practice-management/digital/5-huge-ways-pandemic-has-changed-telemedicine

Federal Changes, State Actions, and Future Policy Considerations

https://www.commonwealthfund.org/publications/issue-briefs/2021/jun/states-actions-expand-telemedicine-access-covid-19

https://www.healio.com/news/primary-care/20201210/cms-makes-some-telehealth-services-permanent-after-covid19

Chapter Links

Chapter 1:

In the beginning: http://www.liebertpub.com/overview/history-of-telemedicine/317/

Department of Agriculture: https://www.rd.usda.gov/programs-services/distance-learning-telemedicine-grants

cellular access: http://www.pewinternet.org/fact-sheet/mobile/

COVID's Impact: https://www.mckinsey.com/industries/healthcare-systems-and-services/our-insights/telehealth-a-quarter-trillion-dollar-post-covid-19-reality

"up to $250 billion of US Healthcare spend could potentially be shifted to virtual or virtually enabled care." https://www.mckinsey.com/industries/healthcare-systems-and-services/our-insights/telehealth-a-quarter-trillion-dollar-post-covid-19-reality

Chapter 2

Health Information Technology for Economic and Clinical Health Act (HITECH Act) of 2009: https://www.healthit.gov/policy-researchers-implementers/health-it-legislation

provisions to improve the flow and exchange of electronic health information."
https://www.healthit.gov/topic/laws-regulation-and-policy/health-it-legislation

Medicare withholds payment:
https://www.cms.gov/medicare/medicare-fee-for-service-payment/acuteinpatientpps/readmissions-reduction-program.html

Developed by Don Berwick, Tom Nolan, and John Wittington:
http://www.ihi.org/resources/Pages/IHIWhitePapers/AGuidetoMeasuringTripleAim.aspx

Institute for Healthcare Improvement (IHI):
http://www.ihi.org/Topics/TripleAim/Pages/default.aspx

Between 2000 and 2019, people aged 65 and up increased from 12.4 to 16.5%, with some states like Montana, Florida, and Hawaii already between 19 and 21.2%. Maine has 21.2% of its population at or above 65 years of age.
https://www.prb.org/usdata/indicator/age65/snapshot

Patients with chronic conditions like diabetes and depression and those who have breathing problems or are immunocompromised were much more likely to use telemedicine in 2020.
https://www.kff.org/medicare/issue-brief/medicare-and-telehealth-coverage-and-use-during-the-covid-19-pandemic-and-options-for-the-future/

EMTALA: https://www.acep.org/life-as-a-physician/ethics--legal/emtala/emtala-fact-sheet/#:~:text=The%20Emergency%20Medical%20Treatment%20and,has%20remained%20an%20unfunded%20mandate.

3.3%: https://www.advisory.com/daily-briefing/2017/09/12/ed-visits-avoidable

90 percent of emergency room care is unnecessary or avoidable: https://healthitanalytics.com/news/how-many-emergency-department-visits-are-really-avoidable

has steadily decreased: https://www.forbes.com/sites/brucejapsen/2019/02/18/u-s-primary-care-doctor-supply-has-improved-but-not-everywhere/?sh=1c5090185c6b

To be successful, a family practitioner must see 20 to 24 patients per day: https://www.washingtonpost.com/news/to-your-health/wp/2014/05/22/how-many-patients-should-your-doctor-see-each-day/?utm_term=.6c256db64ded

Physician extenders, like Physician Assistants and Nurse Practitioners, are using telemedicine to monitor chronic patients. https://www.fiercehealthcare.com/practices/primary-care-using-nps-and-pas-to-reach-patients-virtual-visits reversing the trend of the primary care physician as the center of a family: https://www.reuters.com/article/us-health-pcp-trends-idUSKBN1YK1Z4

It is estimated that 17-42% of patients are "un-doctored," meaning they do not have a primary care physician who manages their care: http://www.fiercehealthcare.com/practices/many-americans-don-t-have-a-primary-care-doctor

the consumer with choices: https://www.pcpcc.org/2019/03/12/patients-consumers

consumer: https://www.sehealthcarequalityconsulting.com/2019/01/11/consumer-driven-trends-in-the-patient-experience/#:~:text=%20Consumer-Driven%20Trends%20in%20the%20Patient%20Experience%20,Protection%20and%20Affordable%20Care%20Act%20in...%20More%20

the retail pharmacies started capitalizing on this trend: https://www.forbes.com/sites/greatspeculations/2015/08/28/walgreens-steps-up-retail-clinic-expansion-as-demand-for-convenient-care-grows/#3faab147141chttp://www.drugchannels.net/2017/02/retail-clinic-check-up-cvs-retrenches.html

Walmart sees a future here, as well, recently purchasing Me MD. https://corporate.walmart.com/newsroom/2021/05/

06/walmart-health-to-acquire-telehealth-provider-memd

As mentioned earlier, specialists reside primarily in urban areas: https://www.ncbi.nlm.nih.gov/pmc/articles/PMC1071163/

As patients become increasingly comfortable using technology, cell phone use improves, and broadband access: http://www.pewresearch.org/fact-tank/2016/07/12/28-of-americans-are-strong-early-adopters-of-technology/

rural areas https://www.pewresearch.org/fact-tank/2019/05/31/digital-gap-between-rural-and-nonrural-america-persists/

Department of Health and Human Services has significantly expanded the support for rural areas. They also instituted flexible provisions to support telemedicine in rural areas. Some of the provisions include: https://www.hhs.gov/coronavirus/telehealth/index.html

CHAPTER 3

Specifically, telehealth is the exchange of medical information between one site and another with the objective to provide medical care, consultation, or

education using information technology:
http://www.himss.org/introduction-telehealth

to the use of mobile technology and wireless devices to improve health outcomes, deliver healthcare services and health research. (HIMSS):
http://www.himss.org/definitions-mhealth

CHAPTER 4

No links

CHAPTER 5

American Health Association:
https://www.heart.org/idc/groups/heart-public/@wcm/@adv/documents/downloadable/ucm_473486.pdf
American Stroke Association:
http://www.stroke.org/we-can-help/healthcare-professionals/improve-your-skills/guide-telestroke
Genentech: https://www.gene.com/medical-professionals/medicines/activase
There are only 28,000 psychiatrists, nationwide:
https://www.forbes.com/sites/brucejapsen/2018/02/25/psychiatrist-shortage-escalates-as-u-s-mental-health-needs-grow/?sh=43c7d0812554

Low acuity urgent care visits:
https://www.wsj.com/articles/with-direct-primary-care-its-just-doctor-and-patient-1488164702
By some estimates, in 2018, teleurgent care visits are already exceeding 1.2 million annually, resulting in significant savings.:
http://www.hhnmag.com/articles/8350-telehealth-adoption-to-double-by-2018&
like Cigna purchasing MD Live:
https://www.fiercehealthcare.com/payer/cigna-s-evernorth-completes-acquisition-virtual-care-provider-mdlive#:~:text=Cigna's%20Evernorth%20has%20completed%20its,efforts%20to%20lower%20healthcare%20costs.

CHAPTER 6

A report by the Kaiser Family Foundation found that 30 to 67 percent of hospitalizations among SNF residents could be prevented with well-targeted interventions.:
http://kaiserfamilyfoundation.files.wordpress.com/2013/01/8109.pdf

widespread opioid use:
https://www.samhsa.gov/data/sites/default/files/reports/rpt29393/2019NSDUHFFRPDFWHTML/2019NSDUHFFR1PDFW090120.pdf
Using telemedicine allows:
https://www.healio.com/news/primary-care/20200211/medicationassisted-therapy-via-telemedicine-shows-promise
One:
https://www.healio.com/news/psychiatry/20170203/telepsychiatry-inperson-mat-comparable-for-opioid-addiction
The federal government agrees.:
https://www.healio.com/news/psychiatry/20161023/video-behavioral-interventions-medication-assisted-treatment-key-to-treating-opioid-addiction
Kaiser Family Foundation white paper:
https://www.kff.org/medicare/issue-brief/medicare-and-telehealth-coverage-and-use-during-the-covid-19-pandemic-and-options-for-the-future/
study showed a greater "mean reduction in hemoglobin A1c":
https://www.endocrinologyadvisor.com/home/topics

/diabetes/telemedicine-for-diabetes-management-update-and-interviews/
the rates are rising exponentially:
https://www.diabetesatlas.org/en/sections/worldwide-toll-of-diabetes.html
Washington University Physicians proves this use case is viable.: https://fertility.wustl.edu/treatments-services/telemedicine/
Called Telehealth ROCKS (Rural Outreach for the Children of Kansas):
http://www.kumc.edu/community-engagement/ku-center-for-telemedicine-and-telehealth/project-echo/telehealth-rocks.html
An important double-blind placebo-controlled study:
https://www.ncbi.nlm.nih.gov/pubmed/11761593
Banner Health's eICU program has saved lives while reducing costs and preserving resources
http://telemedicine.arizona.edu/blog/banner-health-eicu-shortens-hospital-stays-improves-patient-care
Utah Valley Regional Medical Center in Provo, Utah, collaborated with VSee, to support the 60-bed NICU:
http://www.healthcareitnews.com/news/utah-hospital-nicu-goes-virtual-touts-telemedicine-redesign

Studies have shown remote patient monitoring reduces unnecessary emergency department usage by 25–50 percent: http://www.beckershospitalreview.com/healthcare-information-technology/5-top-reasons-why-remote-patient-monitoring-is-destined-to-take-off.html
Cardiology: https://intouchhealth.com/telehealth-solutions/cardiology/
Dermatology: https://www.ama-assn.org/practice-management/digital/teledermatology-paved-way-permanente-s-telehealth-transformation
Thoracic: https://www.infoway-inforoute.ca/en/what-we-do/blog/174-what-we-do/digital-health-and-you/stories/clinician-stories/67-a-thoracic-surgeon-talks-about-the-benefits-of-telemedicine

CHAPTER 7
Project ECHO: http://echo.unm.edu/

Project ECHO operates more than 203 hubs in the US, 423 global hubs, and 920 ECHO programs in 44 countries.: https://hsc.unm.edu/echo/data-marketplace/interactive-dashboards/

CHAPTER 8

DHHS waivers:
https://www.hhs.gov/coronavirus/telehealth/index.html

CHAPTER 9

CMS billing guidelines:
https://www.cms.gov/Medicare/Medicare-General-Information/Telehealth/Telehealth-Codes

Johns Hopkins:
http://www.hopkinsmedicine.org/second_opinion/index.html

CHAPTER 10

there were significant changes made during the pandemic: https://www.cms.gov/newsroom/fact-sheets/medicare-telemedicine-health-care-provider-fact-sheet
https://www.cms.gov/newsroom/fact-sheets/medicare-telemedicine-health-care-provider-fact-sheet

Health Professional Shortage Area:
https://datawarehouse.hrsa.gov/tools/analyzers/hpsa
find.aspx

CHAPTER 11

Teladoc merged with Livongo and purchased
InTouch:
https://hitconsultant.net/2020/12/31/2020-digital-
health-mergers-acquisitions-deals/#.YRBBV4hKiUk

BlueCross/Blue Shield of MDLive:
https://www.bcbstx.com/find-care/providers-in-
your-network/virtual-visit
Large electronic health record (EHR) technology
vendors: https://ehrintelligence.com/news/what-are-
the-top-telehealth-ehr-integrations-in-healthcare
Philips:
http://www.usa.philips.com/healthcare/product/HC
NOCTN503/eicu-program-telehealth-for-the-
intensive-care-unit
Hicuity Health: https://www.advancedicucare.com
In Touch Health: https://www.intouchhealth.com
Specialists on Call:
https://www.specialistsoncall.com

VSee: https://vsee.com
eVisit: https://www.evisit.com
American Well: https://www.americanwell.com
Zoom: https://www.zoom.us/healthcare
Doctor on Demand:
https://www.doctorondemand.com
Teladoc: https://www.teladoc.com
Mend: https://www.mend.com
Doxy.me: https://www.doxy.me
AMC Health: https://www.amchealth.com
Global Med: https://www.globalmed.com

CHAPTER 12

No links

CHAPTER 13

conducting telemedicine encounters is critical.
https://www.hopkinsmedicine.org/office-of-johns-hopkins-physicians/education-training/telemedicine.html

resisters and tailoring the communications to them:
https://www.gartner.com/en/corporate-communications/insights/change-communication

Risk:
https://www.ashrm.org/sites/default/files/ashrm/TELEMEDICINE-WHITE-PAPER.pdf

The American Society for Health Care Risk Management has an excellent whitepaper addressing telemedicine:
https://www.ashrm.org/sites/default/files/ashrm/TELEMEDICINE-WHITE-PAPER.pdf
Workflows: https://digital.ahrq.gov/health-it-tools-and-resources/evaluation-resources/workflow-assessment-health-it-toolkit/workflow

CHAPTER 14

legal, safe harbors:
https://mhealthintelligence.com/news/stark-law-changes-should-benefit-telehealth-remote-patient-monitoring
According to one attorney:
https://nixongwiltlaw.com/nlg-blog/2020/11/22/changes-to-the-anti-kickback-regulations-are-good-news-for-digital-health-innovation-and-the-shift-to-value-based-care

"Standards for Privacy of Individually Identifiable Health Information," issued by the Department of Health and Human Services (HHS). https://aspe.hhs.gov/standards-privacy-individually-identifiable-health-information

its Senate report 111-66.: https://www.congress.gov/congressional-report/111th-congress/senate-report/66

here. : https://fsmb.org/siteassets/advocacy/pdf/states-waiving-licensure-requirements-for-telehealth-in-response-to-covid-19.pdf

CHAPTER 15

Federation of State Medical Boards: https://www.fsmb.org/

"An interstate compact is a legal agreement among participating states that allows them to work closely together to address issues of mutual concern that cross state borders. Hundreds of compacts exist in the United States, and they have helped states address everything from shared water use to transportation issues.

In the case of the Interstate Medical Licensure Compact, it is an agreement that allows states to work together to significantly streamline the licensing process for physicians who want to practice in multiple states.”: https://www.imlcc.org/faqs/

the Interstate Medical Licensure Compact: http://www.imlcc.org/
FSMB: https://www.fsmb.org/
IMLC: https://www.imlcc.org/

CHAPTER 16

No links

Biography

Ms. Kamenca has been deeply involved in healthcare services, including serving as an executive director for a medical research organization associated with the Veterans Administration, an executive for a non-profit public health organization, and directing telemedicine services for two large hospital systems. For one large health system, she managed all aspects of the Arizona telemedicine solutions and then was promoted to initiate telehealth projects for the corporate enterprise. Her key telehealth projects included video visits, teleradiology and image transfer solutions, secure messaging, remote patient monitoring, telepsychiatry, rural telemedicine implementations, and other clinical innovation projects (like Google Glass for physician productivity.) At a separate health system, she directed their rural telehealth initiative and developed their eVisit program.

Ms. Kamenca's background includes growing key business initiatives for a large pharmaceutical company, IBM, PriceWaterhouseCoopers, and a Microsoft Solutions partner. She started and grew a small business that delivered consulting services to organizations including

Allied Waste, Maricopa County, the Arizona Department of Transportation, and the City of Phoenix.

Ms. Kamenca earned a Master of Business Administration from the University of Southern California, where she was a Simonsen Fellow. She also earned a post-graduate Certificate in Healthcare Informatics from the University of Colorado, Denver.

MindView Press

Printed in the United States
Ebook: ISBN-13: 978-1-949761-89-4
Paperback: ISBN-13: 978-1-949761-91-7

Made in the USA
Las Vegas, NV
22 August 2022

53776749R00095